# ANATOMY AND PHYSIOLOGY

## COLORING BOOK

**ANATOMY DISTRICT**

If you would like to show your support, we would greatly appreciate a rating and review on Amazon. Please scan this QR with your smarpthone's camera and you will be directed to the reviews section. Thank you!

# TABLE OF CONTENTS

# TABLE OF CONTENTS

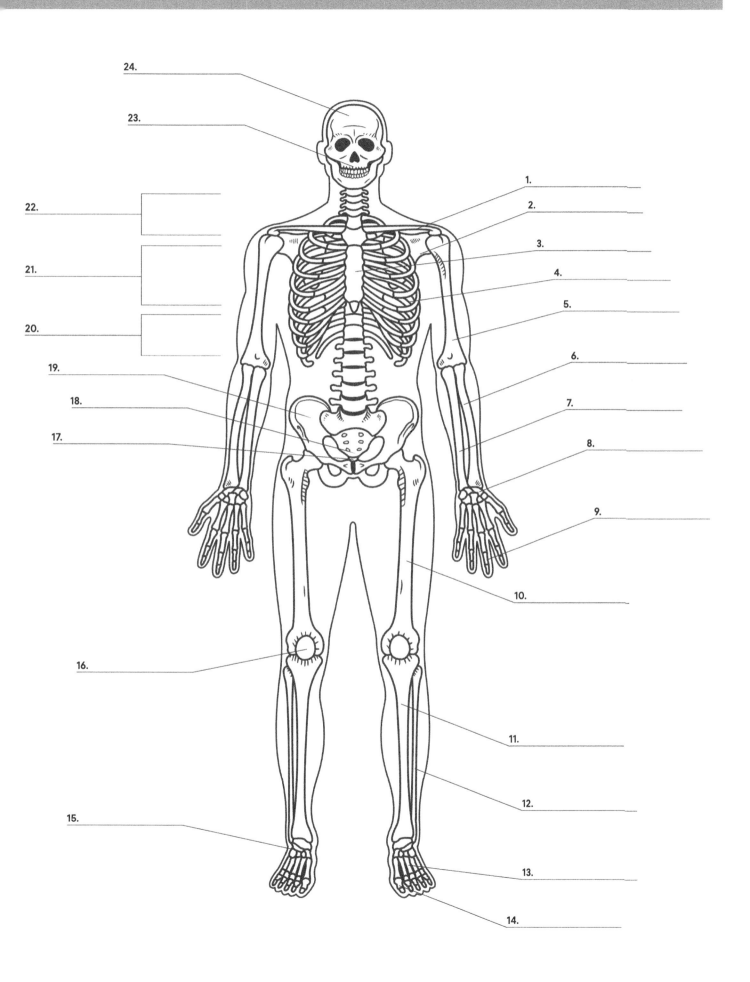

1. Clavicle
2. Scapula
3. Sternum
4. Ribs
5. Humerus
6. Radius
7. Ulna
8. Metacarpals
9. Phalanges
10. Femur
11. Tibia
12. Fibula
13. Metarsals
14. Phalanges
15. Tarsals
16. Patella
17. Coccyx
18. Sacrum
19. Pelvis
20. Lumbar vertebrae
21. Thoracic vertebrae
22. Cervical vertebrae
23. Mandible
24. Skull

## NOTES:

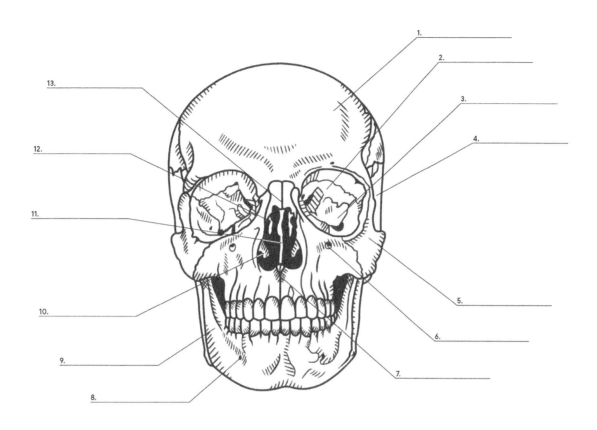

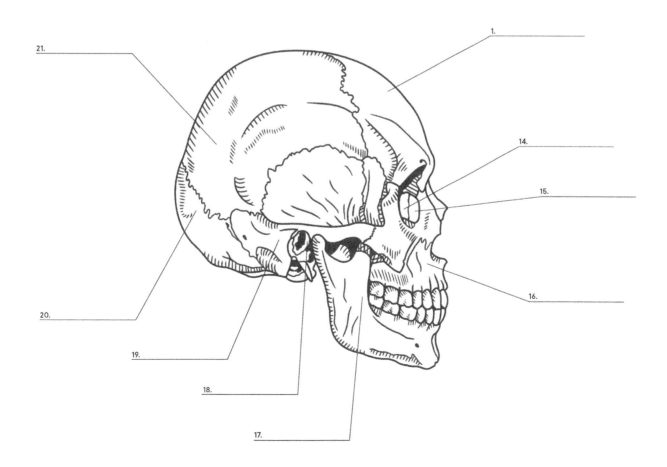

1. Frontal Bone
2. Sphenoid bone (lesser wing)
3. Sphenoid bone (greater wing)
4. Temporal bone
5. Zygomatic bone
6. Intraorbital foramen
7. Anterior nasal spine
8. Mental foramen
9. Ramus
10. Inferior nasal concha
11. Vomer
12. Middle nasal concha
13. Nasal bone
14. Ethmoid bone
15. Lacrimal bone
16. Maxilla
17. Mandible
18. External acoustic meatus
19. Temporal bone
20. Occipital bone
21. Parietal bone

NOTES:

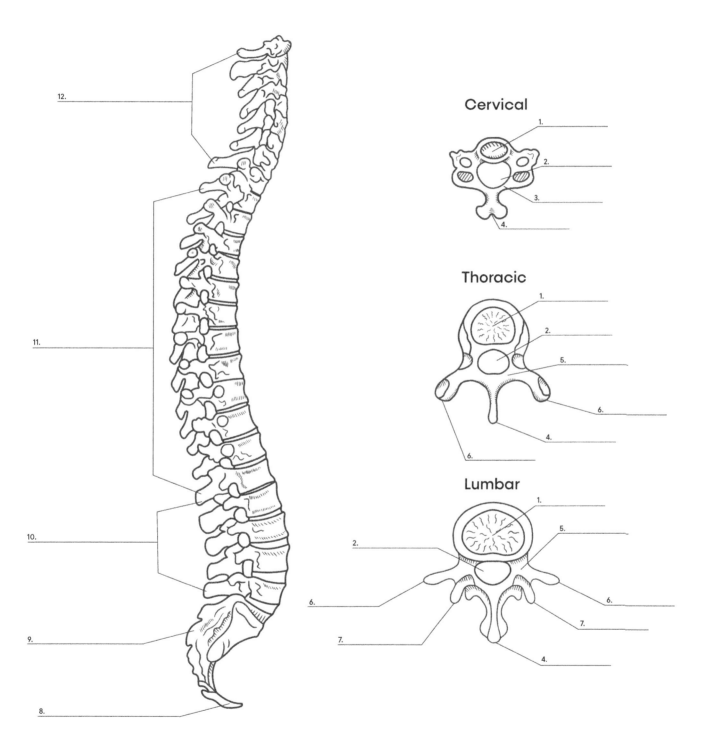

Cervical

1.
2.
3.
4.

Thoracic

1.
2.
5.
6.
4.
6.

Lumbar

1.
2.
5.
6.
7.
7.
4.

12.
11.
10.
9.
8.

1. Body
2. Vertebral foramen
3. Ars
4. Spinous process
5. Lamina
6. Transverse process

7. Articular process
8. Coccyx
9. Sacrum
10. Lumbar
11. Thoracic
12. Cervical

## NOTES:

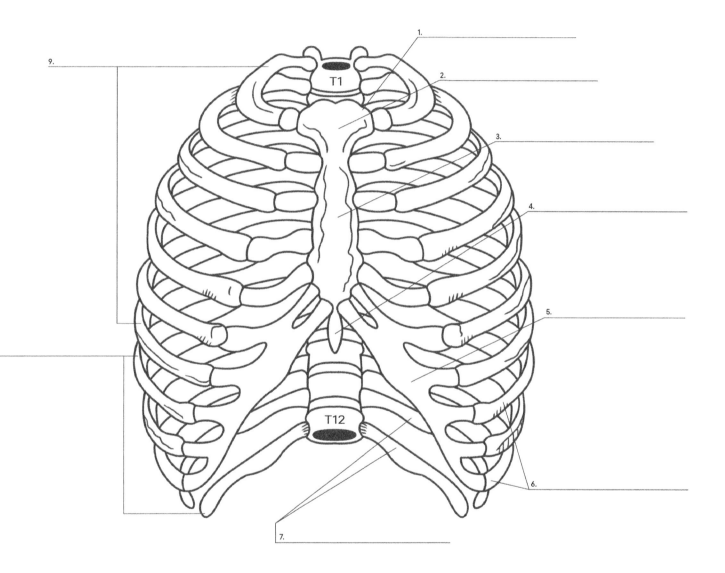

1.

2.

3.

4.

5.

6.

7.

9.

T1

T12

# 1.d. SKELETAL SYSTEM - RIBS ANATOMY

1. Clavicular articulation
2. Manubrium ( Sternum)
3. Body (Sternum)
4. Xiphoid process ( Sternum)
5. Costal cartilage
6. Vertebrochondral ( Ribs 8-10)
7. Floating ribs ( Ribs 11-12)
8. False ribs ( Ribs 8-12)
9. True ribs ( Vertebrosterenal) (Ribs 1-7)

## NOTES:

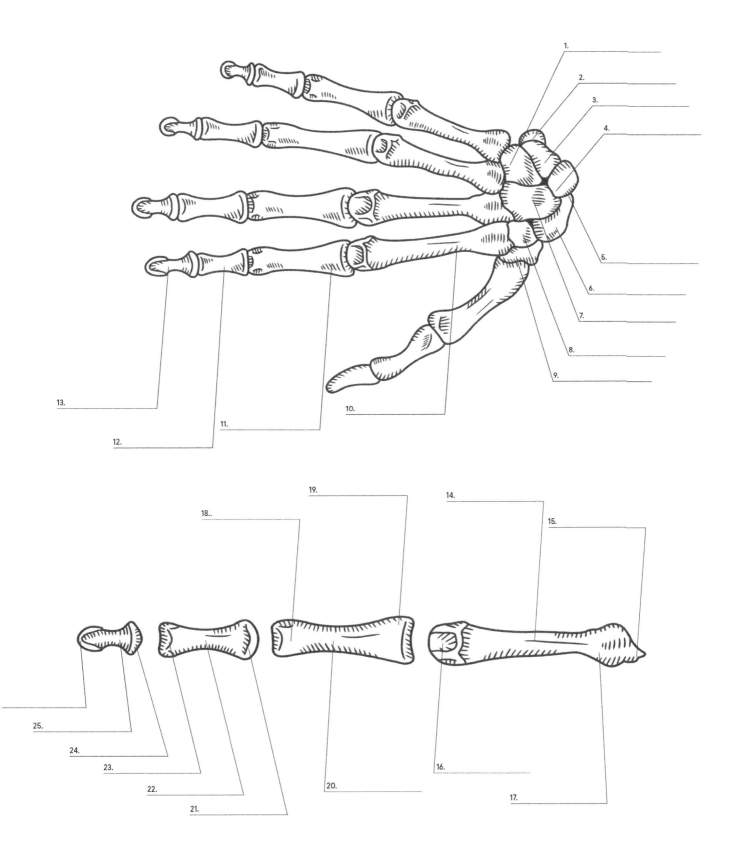

1. Hamatum bone
2. Piriform bone
3. Triquetrum bone
4. Lunatum bone
5. Carpus
6. Scaphoid bone
7. Capitatum bone
8. Multangulum minus bone
9. Multangulum majus bone
10. Metacarpal
11. Proximal phalanx
12. Middle phalanx
13. Distal phalanx

14. Corpus
15. Styloideus Process
16. Capitulum
17. Basis
18. Trochlea
19. Basis
20. Corpus
21. Basis
22. Trochlear Body
23. Trochlea
24. Basis
25. Corpus
26. Tuberosity of distal phalanx

## NOTES:

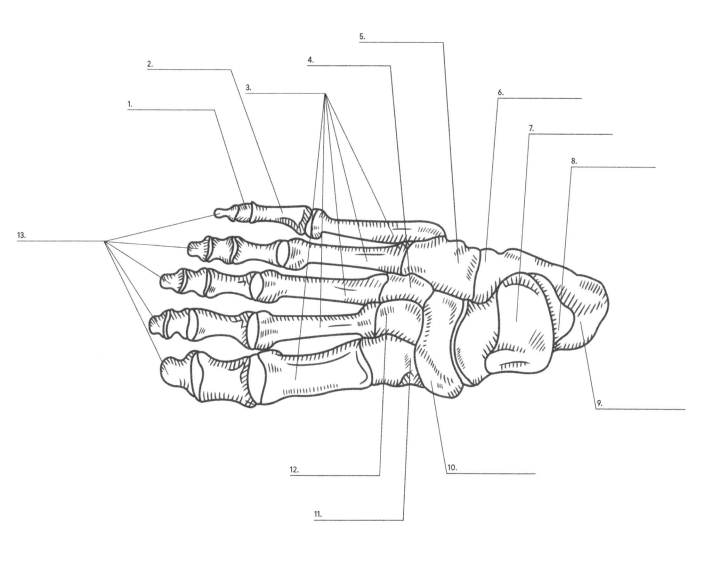

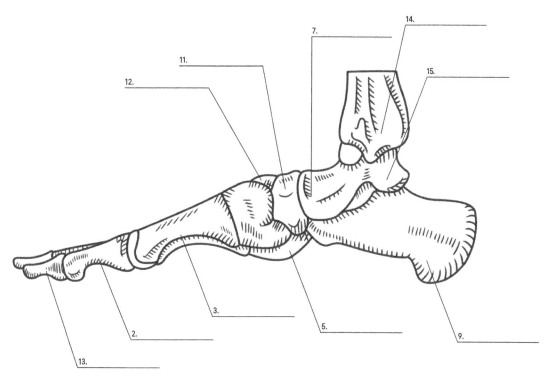

1. Middle phalanx
2. Proximal phalangs
3. Metatarsals
4. Lateral cuneiform
5. Cuboid bone
6. Calcaneus
7. Talus bone
8. Processus posterior

9. Calcaneus tuber
10. Navicular
11. Medial cuneiform
12. Intermediate cuneiform
13. Distal phalanx
14. Tibia
15. Medial tudercle

## NOTES:

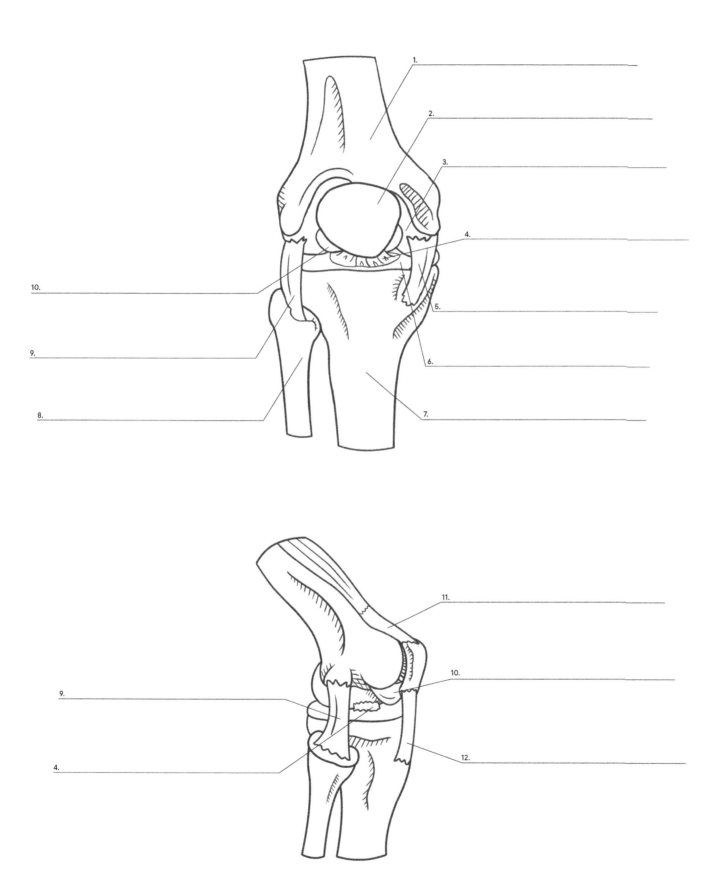

1. _____
2. _____
3. _____
4. _____
5. _____
6. _____
7. _____
8. _____
9. _____
10. _____
11. _____
12. _____

1. Femur
2. Patella
3. Articular cartilage
4. Anterior cruciate ligament
5. Medial collateral ligament
6. Meniscus

7. Tibia
8. Fibula
9. Lateral collateral ligament
10. Posterior cruciate ligament
11. Quadriceps tendon
12. Patellar tendon

## NOTES:

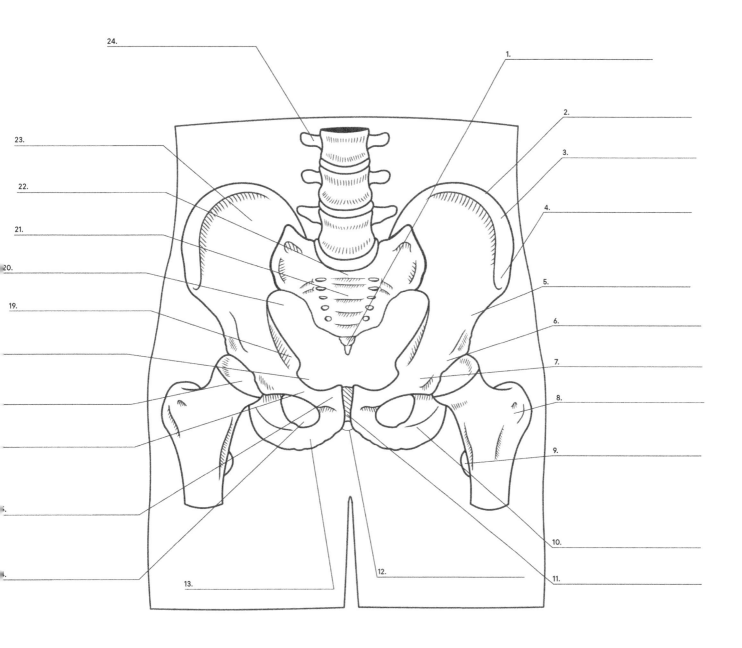

1. Coccyx
2. Iliac crest
3. Tubercle of iliac crest
4. Anterior superior iliac spine
5. Anterior inferior iliac spine
6. Iliopubic eminence
7. Pectineal line
8. Greater trochanter of femur
9. Lesser trochanter of femur
10. Ischial tuberosity
11. Pubic symphysis
12. Pubic arch
13. Inferior pubic ramus
14. Obturator foramen
15. Pubic tubercle
16. Superior pubic ramus
17. Articular cartilage
18. Lesser sciatic notch
19. Ischial spine
20. Greater sciatic notch
21. Sacrum
22. Sacral promontory
23. Wing of ilium
24. Transverse process

NOTES:

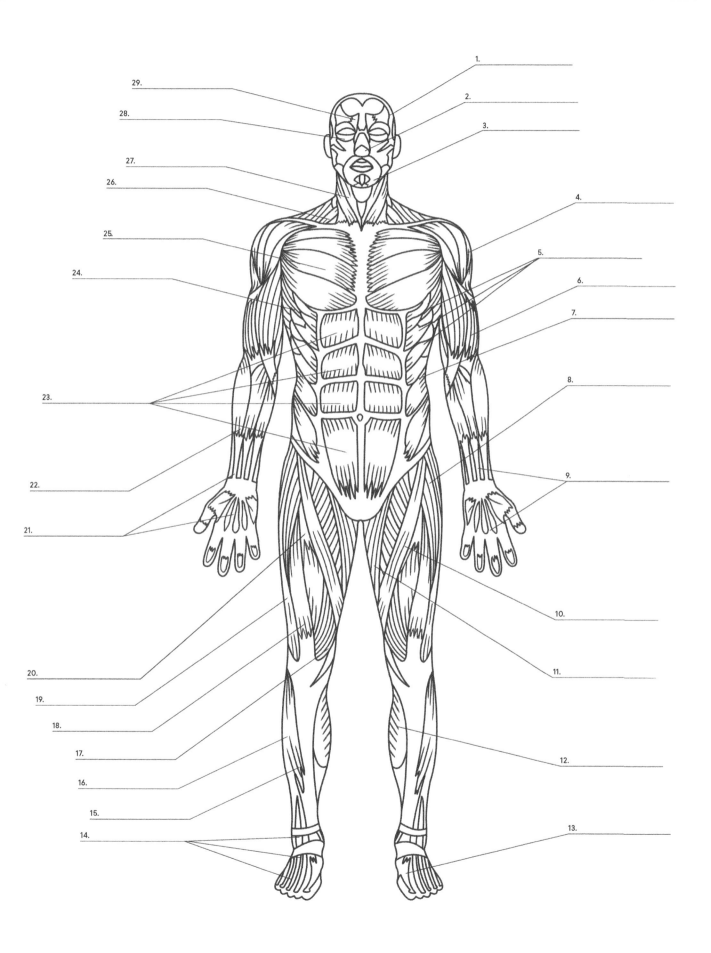

1. Temporalis
2. Nasalis
3. Orbicularis oris
4. Deltoid
5. Serratus anterior
6. Biceps
7. Externus oblique
8. Tensor fascia latae
9. Extenors of the hand
10. Sartorius
11. Adductor lungus
12. Gastrocnemius
13. Flexors of the foot
14. Extensors of the foot
15. Tibialis anterior
16. Peroneus longus
17. Vastus medialis
18. Vastus intermedius
19. Vastus letaralis
20. Recus femoris
21. Flexors of the hand
22. Brachioradialis
23. Rectus abdominis
24. Serratus anterior
25. Pectoralis major
26. Trapezius
27. Sternocleidomastoid
28. Orbicularis oculi
29. Frontalis

## NOTES:

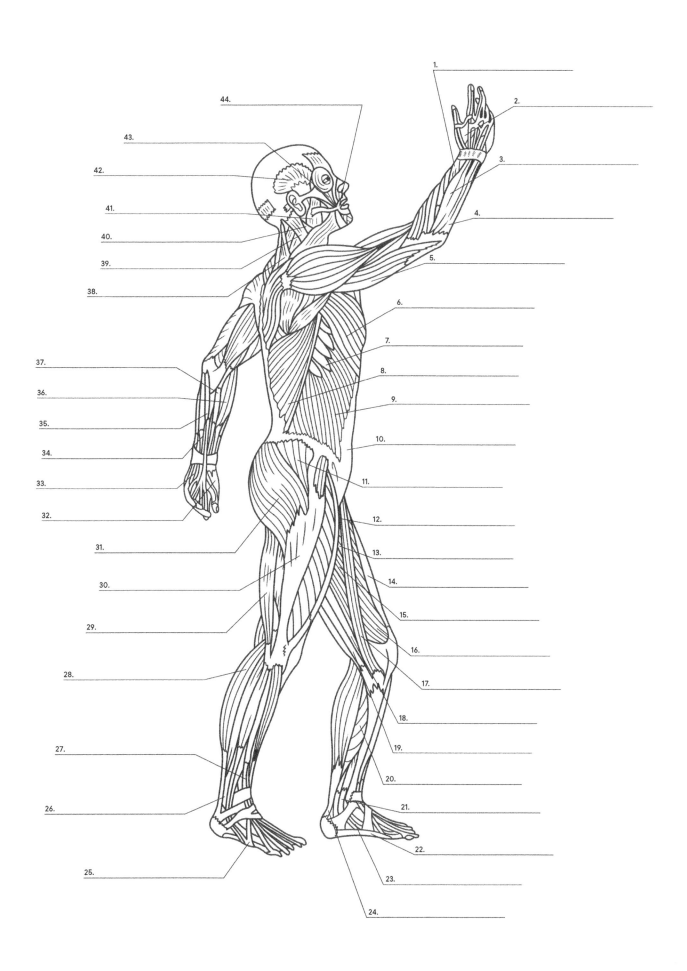

1. _____

2. _____

3. _____

4. _____

5. _____

6. _____

7. _____

8. _____

9. _____

10. _____

11. _____

12. _____

13. _____

14. _____

15. _____

16. _____

17. _____

18. _____

19. _____

20. _____

21. _____

22. _____

23. _____

24. _____

25. _____

26. _____

27. _____

28. _____

29. _____

30. _____

31. _____

32. _____

33. _____

34. _____

35. _____

36. _____

37. _____

38. _____

39. _____

40. _____

41. _____

42. _____

43. _____

44. _____

1. Abductor pollicis longus and extensor pollicis
2. Dorsal introsseous
3. Extensor digitorum
4. Extensor carpi ulnaris
5. Triceps
6. Pectoralis major
7. Serratus anterior
8. Latissimus dorsi
9. Abdomen
10. Rectus abdominis
11. Gluteus medius
12. Iliopsoas
13. Pectineus
14. Rectus femoris
15. Adductor longus
16. Vastus medialis
17. Sartorius
18. Gracilis
19. Semitendinosus
20. Soleus
21. Flexor digitorum and hallucis
22. Short muscles of the sole
23. Tibialis posterior
24. Tendo calcaneus
25. Peroneus tertius
26. Peroneus longus and brevis
27. Extensor digitorum longus
28. Gastrocnemius
29. Biceps femoris
30. Iliotibial tract
31. Gluteus maximus
32. Thenar muscles
33. Hypothenar muscles
34. Flexor digitorum superficialis
35. Palmaris longus
36. Brachioradialis
37. Flexor carpi radialis
38. Trapezius
39. Sternocleidomastoid
40. Digastric and stylohyoid
41. Masseter
42. Temporalis
43. Zygomaticus major
44. Orbicularis oris

## NOTES:

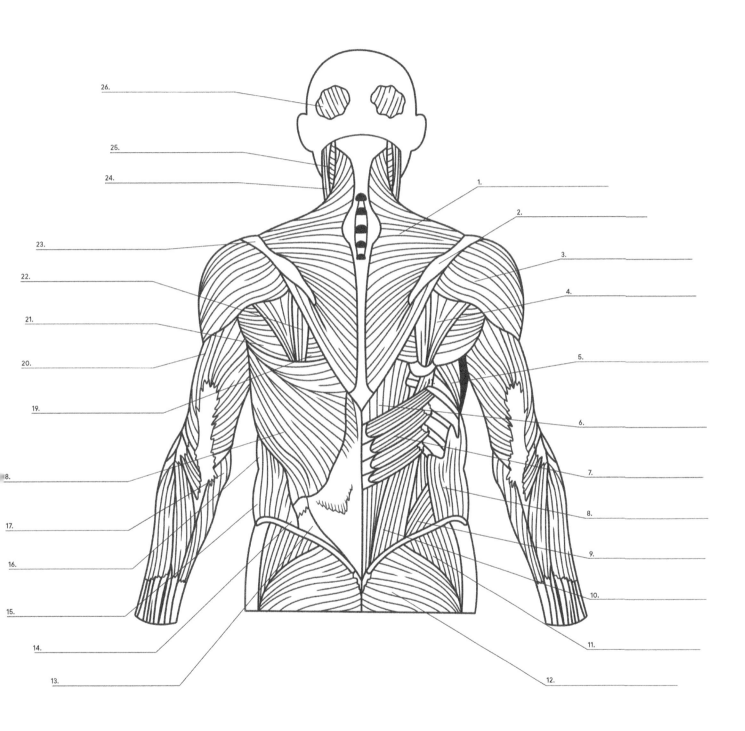

1. Trapezius
2. Acromion
3. Deltoid
4. Scapula inferior angle
5. Serratus anterior
6. Right longissimus thoracis
7. Serratus posterior inferior
8. External oblique
9. Internal oblique
10. Right Iliocostalis lumborum
11. Gluteal Medius
12. Gluteal Maximus
13. Latissimus dorsi

14. Lumbar triangle
15. External oblique abdominal
16. Latissimus dorsi
17. Flexor carpi ulnaris
18. Latissimus dorsi
19. Rhomboid major
20. Triceps
21. Teres major
22. Infraspinatus
23. Spine of scapula
24. Sternocleidomastoid
25. Splenius Capitis
26. Occipitalis

## NOTES:

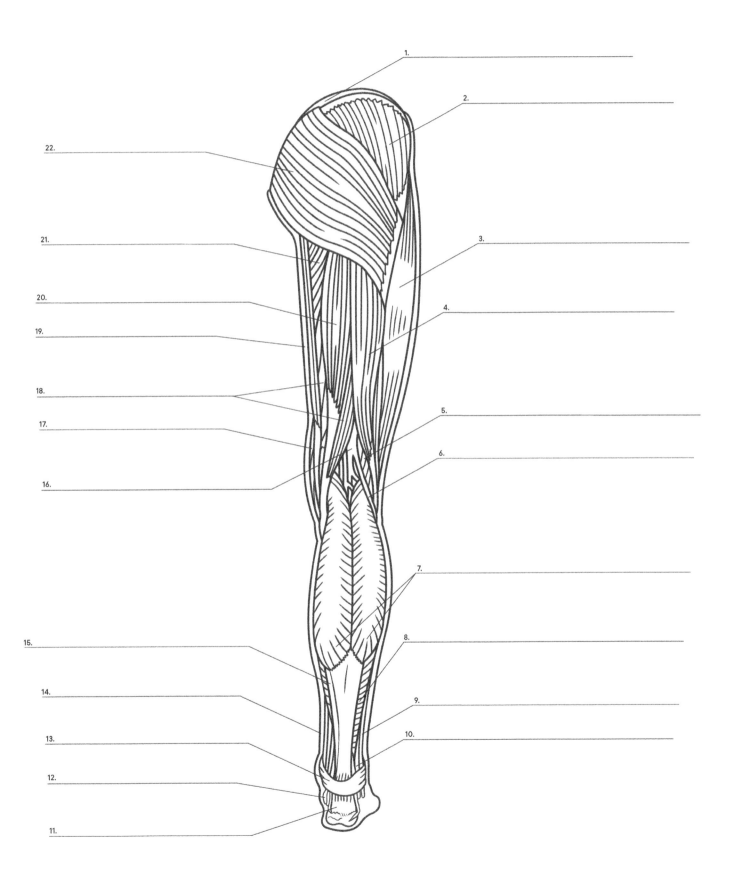

1. _____

2. _____

22. _____

21. _____

3. _____

20. _____

4. _____

19. _____

18. _____

5. _____

17. _____

6. _____

16. _____

7. _____

15. _____

8. _____

14. _____

9. _____

13. _____

10. _____

12. _____

11. _____

1. Iliac crest
2. Gluteus medius muscle
3. Iliotibial tract
4. Biceps femoris muscle
5. Plantaris muscle
6. Comon fibular nerve
7. Gastrocnemius muscle
8. Soleus muscle
9. Fibularis longus tendon
10. Fibularis brevis tendon
11. Flexor hallucis longus tendon
12. Tibial nerve

13. Medial malleolus
14. Flexor digitorum longus tendon
15. Plantaris tendon
16. Tibial nerve
17. Sartorius muscle
18. Semimembranosus muscle
19. Gracilis muscle
20. Semitendinosus
21. Adductor magnus muscle
22. Gluteus maximus muscle

## NOTES:

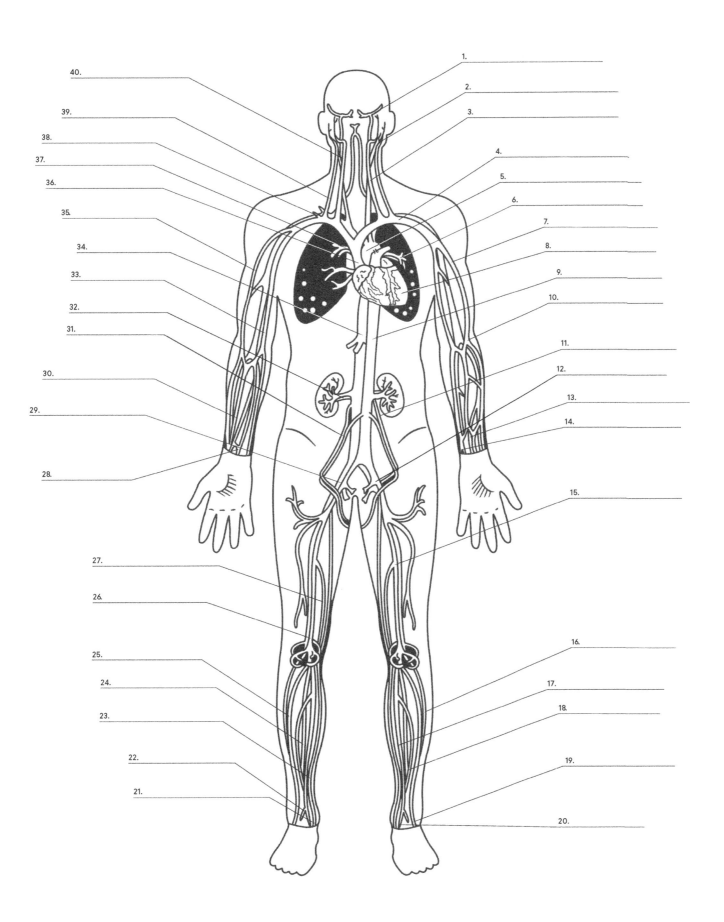

40.

39.

38.

37.

36.

35.

34.

33.

32.

31.

30.

29.

28.

27.

26.

25.

24.

23.

22.

21.

1.

2.

3.

4.

5.

6.

7.

8.

9.

10.

11.

12.

13.

14.

15.

16.

17.

18.

19.

20.

1. Internal carotid artery
2. External carotid artery
3. Common carotid artery
4. Subclavian artery
5. Aorta
6. Pulmonary vein
7. Axillary artery
8. Heart
9. Descending aorta
10. Brachial artery
11. Mesenteric artery
12. Common iliac artery
13. Radial artery
14. Ulnar artery
15. Femoral artery
16. Anterior tibial artery
17. Posterior tibial artery
18. Peroneal artery
19. Arcuate artery
20. Dorsal digital arteries
21. Dorsal digital vein
22. Dorsal venous arch
23. Posterior tibial vein
24. Anterior tibial vein
25. Small saphenous vein
26. Femoral vein
27. Great saphenous vein
28. Palmar digital veins
29. Common iliac vein
30. Medial cubital vein
31. Hepatic portal vein
32. Renal artery
33. Basilic vein
34. Hepatic vein
35. Cephalic vein
36. Superior vena cava
37. Pulmonary artery
38. Subclavian vein
39. External jugular vein
40. Internal jugular vein

## NOTES:

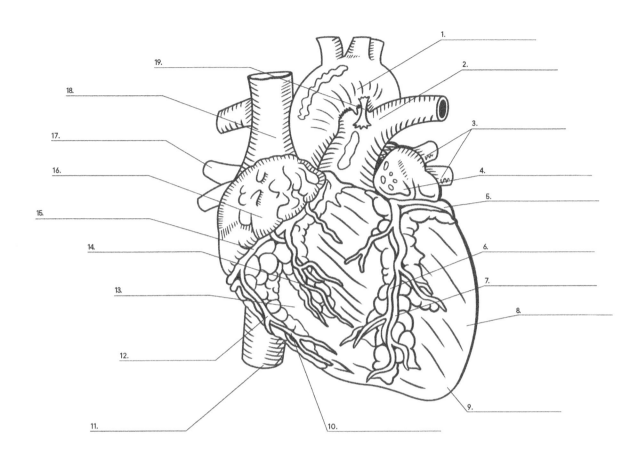

1.
2.
3.
4.
5.
6.
7.
8.
9.
10.
11.
12.
13.
14.
15.
16.
17.
18.
19.

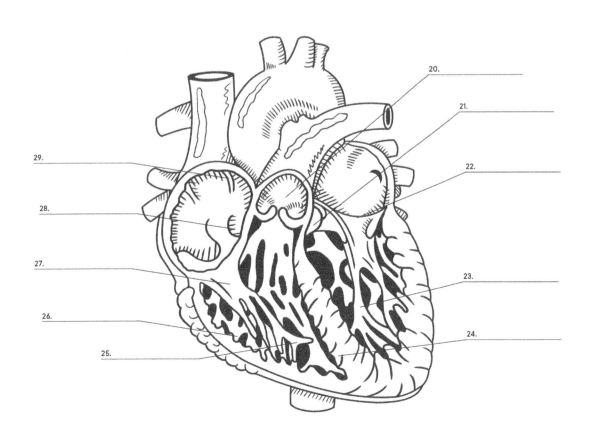

20.
21.
22.
23.
24.
25.
26.
27.
28.
29.

1. Aorta
2. Pulmonary trunk
3. Pulmonary veins
4. Auricle
5. Circumflex artery
6. Great cardiac vein
7. Anterior interventricular artery
8. Left ventricle
9. Apex
10. Small cardiac vein
11. Inferior vena cava
12. Marginal artery
13. Right ventricle
14. Anterior cardiac vein
15. Right coronary artery
16. Right atrium
17. Right pulmonary veins
18. Superior vena cava
19. Ligamentum arteriosum
20. Pulmonary semilunar valve
21. Aortic valve
22. Bicuspid valve
23. Papillary muscle
24. Interventricular septum
25. Chordae tendineae
26. Trabeculae carneae
27. Tricuspid valve
28. Fossa ovalis
29. Sino-atrial node

NOTES:

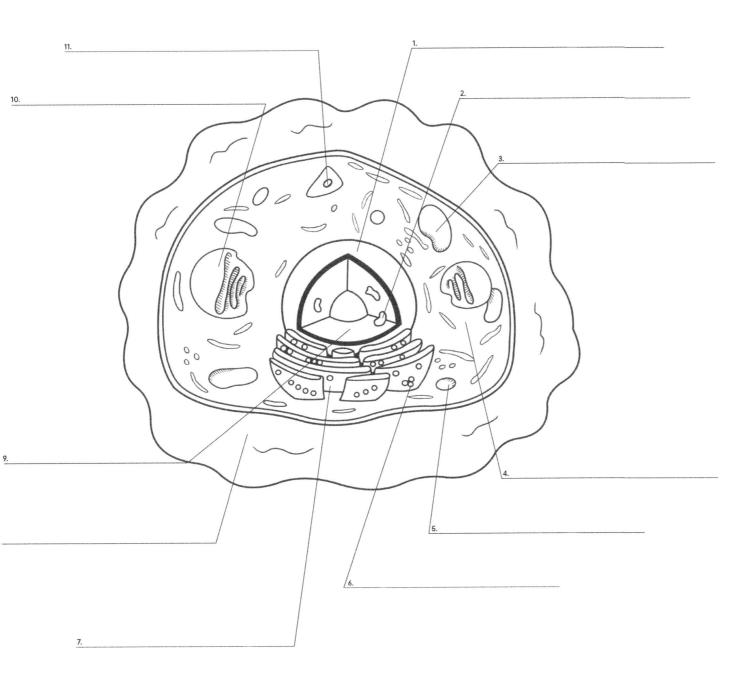

11.

10.

1.

2.

3.

9.

4.

5.

6.

7.

# 4. HUMAN CELL ANATOMY

1. Nuclear membrane
2. Chromosome
3. Mitochondrion
4. Cytoplasm
5. Peroxisome
6. Ribosomes

7. Endoplasmic reticulum
8. Cell membrane
9. Nucleus
10. Golgi bodies
11. Lysosome

## NOTES:

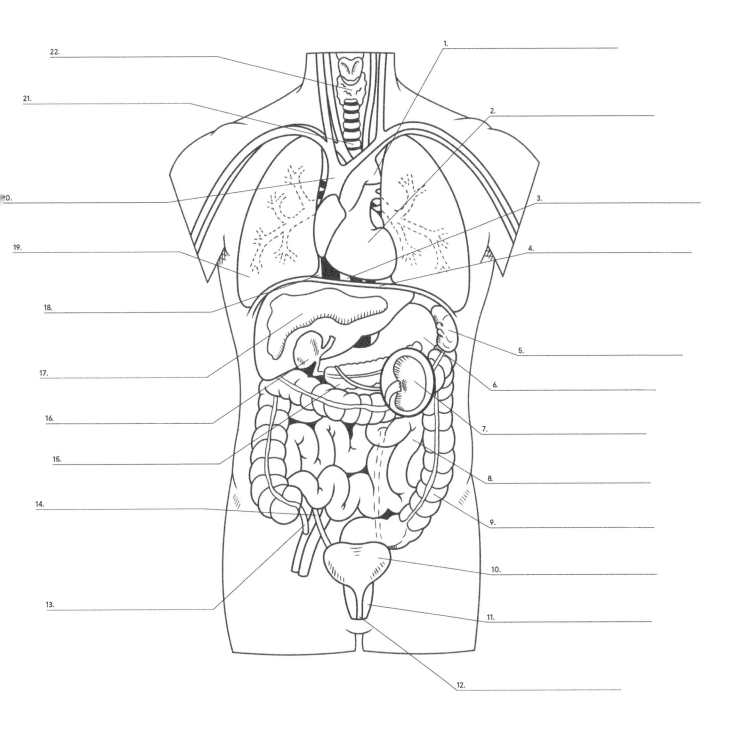

22. _____

21. _____

20. _____

19. _____

18. _____

17. _____

16. _____

15. _____

14. _____

13. _____

1. _____

2. _____

3. _____

4. _____

5. _____

6. _____

7. _____

8. _____

9. _____

10. _____

11. _____

12. _____

1. Aorta
2. Heart
3. Esophagus
4. Diaphragn
5. Spleen
6. Stomach
7. Kidney
8. Small intestine
9. Large intestine
10. Bladder
11. Rectum
12. Urethra

13. Appendix
14. Ureter
15. Pancreas
16. Gallbladder
17. Liver
18. Inferior vena cava
19. Lung
20. Superior vena cava
21. Trachea
22. Thyroid

## NOTES:

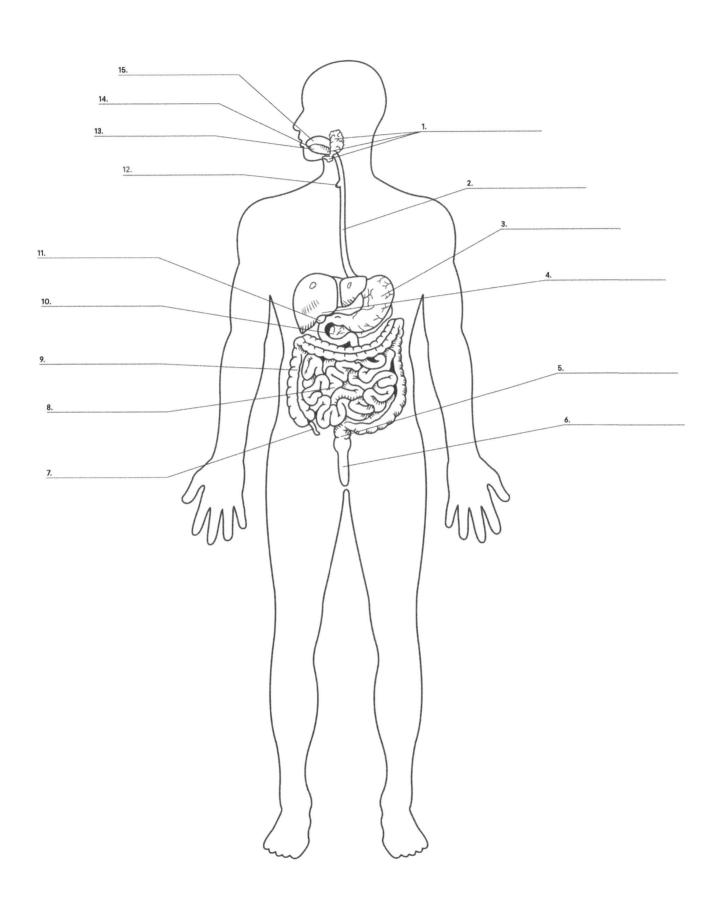

# 6.a. DIGESTIVE SYSTEM - FULL BODY DIAGRAM

1. Salivary glands
2. Esophagus
3. Stomach
4. Liver
5. Rectum
6. Anus
7. Appendix
8. Small Intestine

9. Large instestine
10. Pancreas
11. Gallbladder
12. Epiglottis
13. Tongue
14. Teeth
15. Mouth

## NOTES:

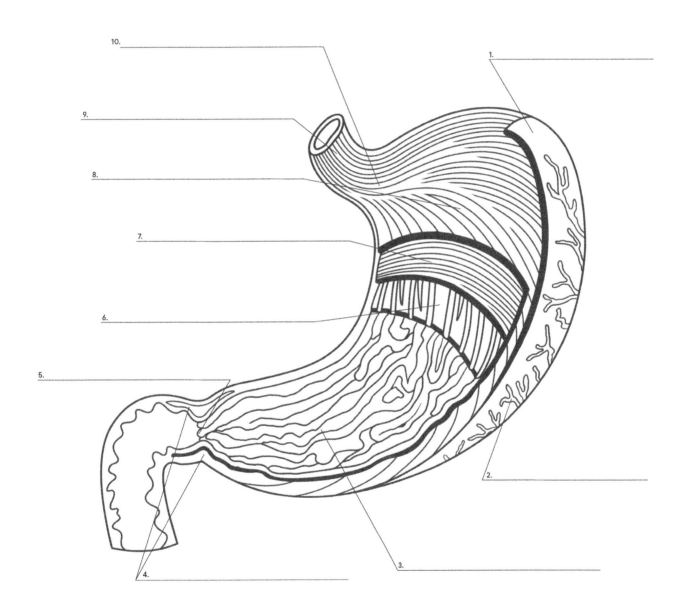

10.

9.

8.

7.

6.

5.

1.

2.

4.

3.

1. Fundus
2. Left gastroepiploic vessels
3. Pyloric antrum
4. Pyloric sphincter
5. Pyloric canal

6. Oblique layer
7. Circular layer
8. Longitudinal layer
9. Esophagus
10. Cardia

## NOTES:

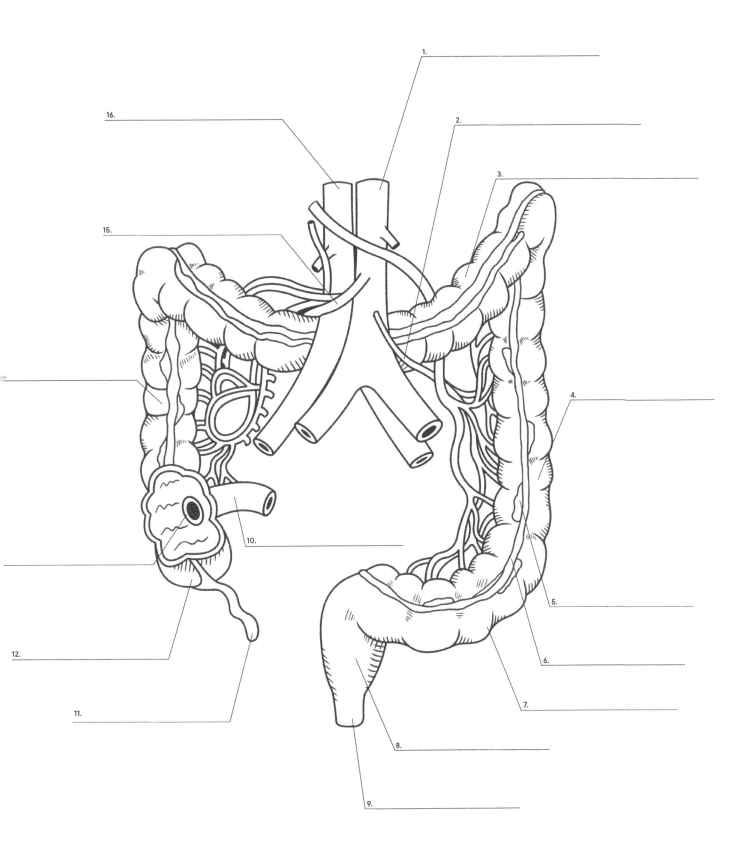

1.

2.

3.

4.

5.

6.

7.

8.

9.

10.

11.

12.

15.

16.

1. Aorta
2. Inferior mesenteric artery
3. Transverse colon
4. Descending colon
5. Fatty appendices
6. Taenia coli
7. Sigmoid colon
8. Rectum
9. Anus
10. Ileum
11. Appendix
12. Cecum
13. Ileocecal valve
14. Ascending colon
15. Superior mesenteric artery
16. Inferior vena cava

**NOTES:**

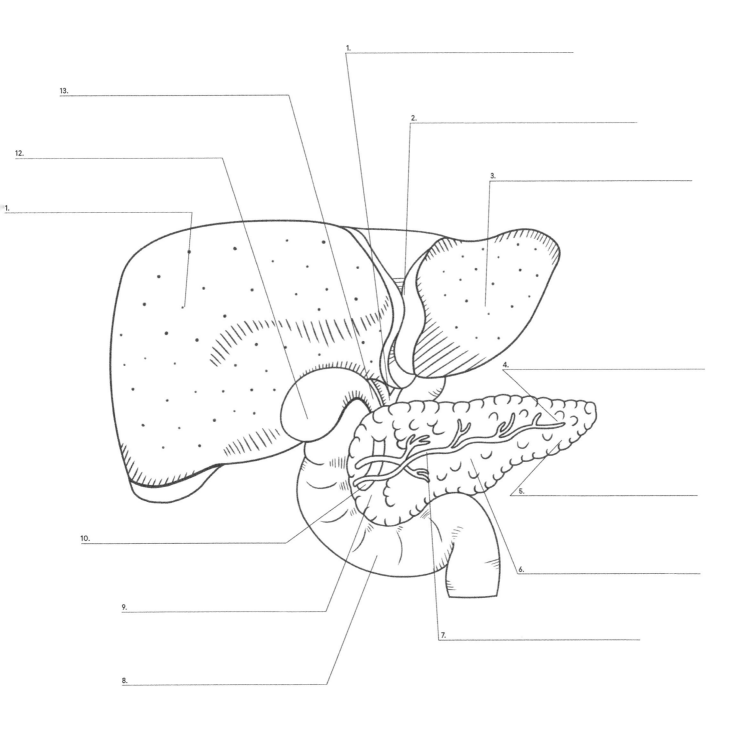

1.

13.

12.

1.

2.

3.

4.

5.

6.

7.

8.

9.

10.

1. Hepatic duct
2. Sulphate ligament
3. Left lobe
4. Tail of pancreas
5. Pancreas
6. Body of pancreas
7. Pancreatic duct

8. Duodenum
9. Head of pancreas
10. Common bile duct
11. Right lobe
12. Gallbladder
13. Cystic duct

## NOTES:

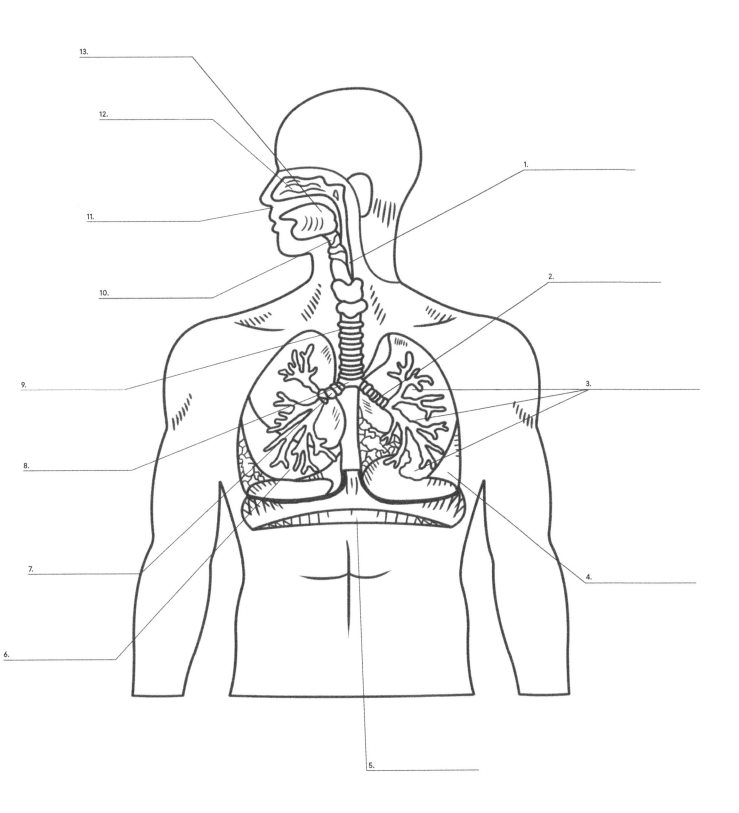

1. Pharynx
2. Left main bronchus
3. Bronchi
4. Left Lung
5. Diaphragm
6. Right lung
7. Right main bronchus

8. Caria of Trachea
9. Trachea
10. Larynx
11. Nostril
12. Nasal Cavity Plus Paranasal Sinuses
13. Oral Cavity

## NOTES:

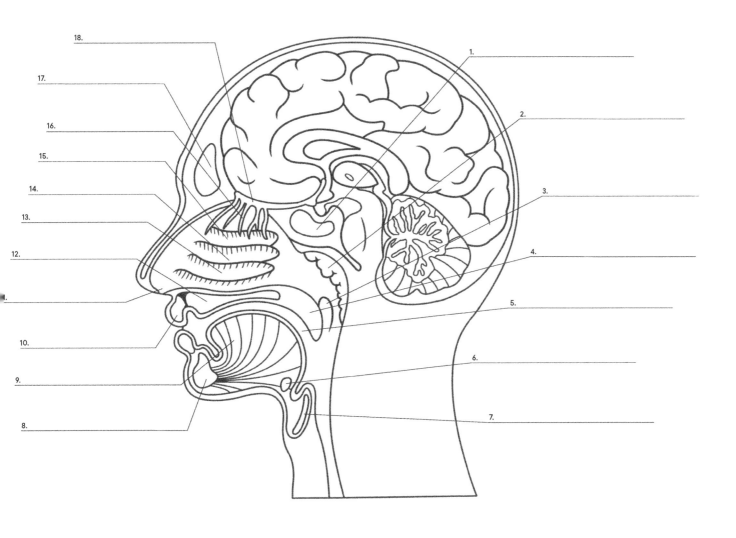

18.

17.

16.

15.

14.

13.

12.

11.

10.

9.

8.

1.

2.

3.

4.

5.

6.

7.

1. Sphenoid sinus
2. Pharingial tonsil
3. Opening of eustachian tube
4. Soft palate
5. Oral cavity
6. Hyoid bone
7. Epiglottis
8. Mandible
9. Tongue
10. Lips
11. Vestibule
12. Hard palate
13. Inferior nasal concha
14. Middle nasal concha
15. Superior nasal concha
16. Olfactory nervs
17. Frontal sinus
18. Olfactory buld

## NOTES:

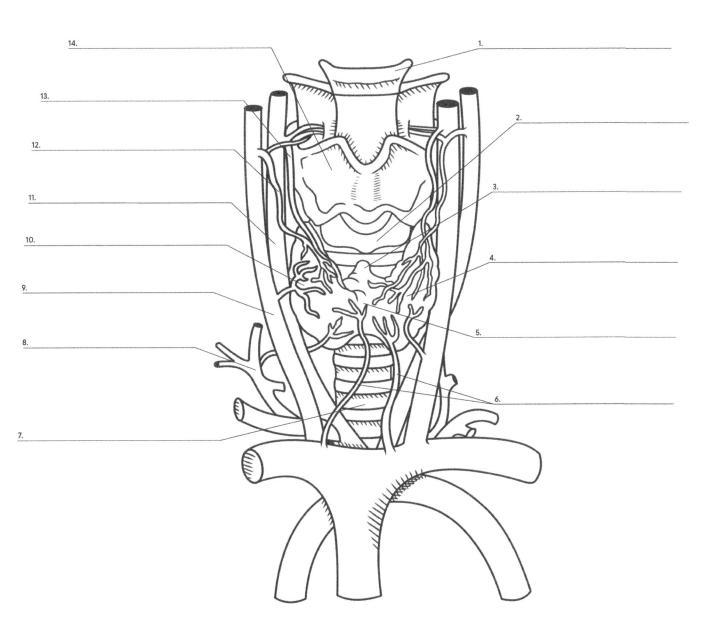

14.

13.

12.

11.

10.

9.

8.

7.

1.

2.

3.

4.

5.

6.

1. Hyoid bone
2. Cricoid cartilage of larynx
3. Pyramidal lobe of thyroid gland
4. Left lobe of thyroid gland
5. Isthmus of thyroid gland
6. Inferior thyroid vein
7. Trachea
8. Inferior thyroid artery
9. Internal Vein
10. Right lobe of thyroid gland
11. Common Carotid artery
12. Superior vein
13. Superior artery
14. Larynx

**NOTES:**

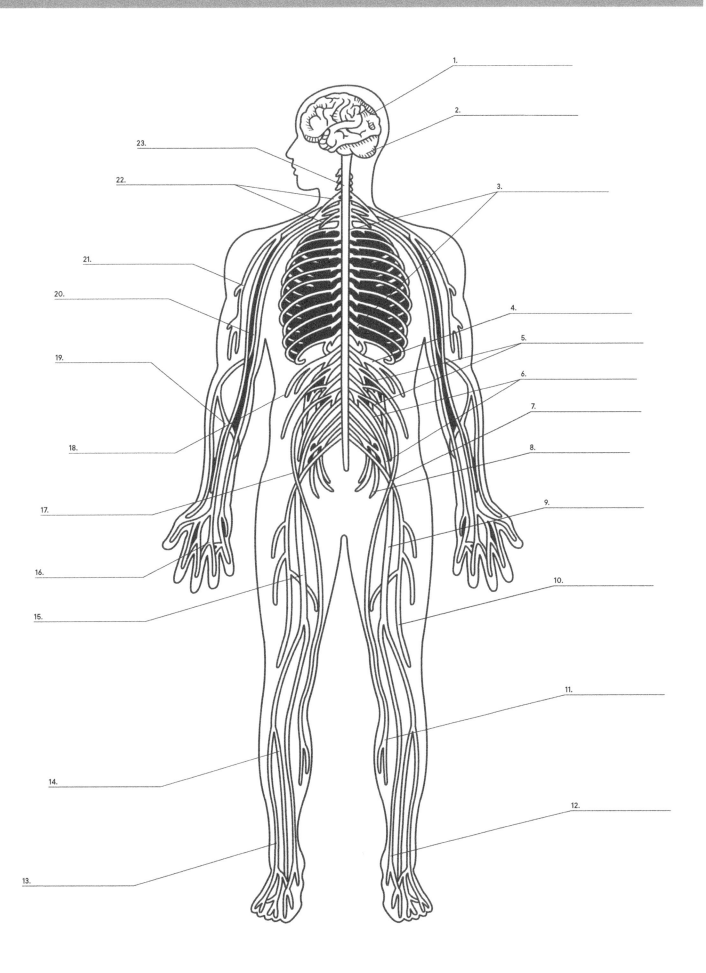

1. Brain
2. Cerebellum
3. Intercostal nerves
4. Subcostal nerve
5. Lumbar plexus
6. Sacral plexus
7. Femoral nerve
8. Pudental nerve
9. Sciatic nerve
10. Muscular branches of femoral nerve
11. Saphenous nerve nerve
12. Tibial nerve
13. Superficial peroneal nerve
14. Deep peroneal nerve
15. Cammon peroneal nerve
16. Ulnar nerve
17. Obturator nerve
18. Illiohypogastric nerve
19. Median nerve
20. Radial nerve
21. Muscolocutaneous nerve
22. Brachial plexus
23. Spinal cord

## NOTES:

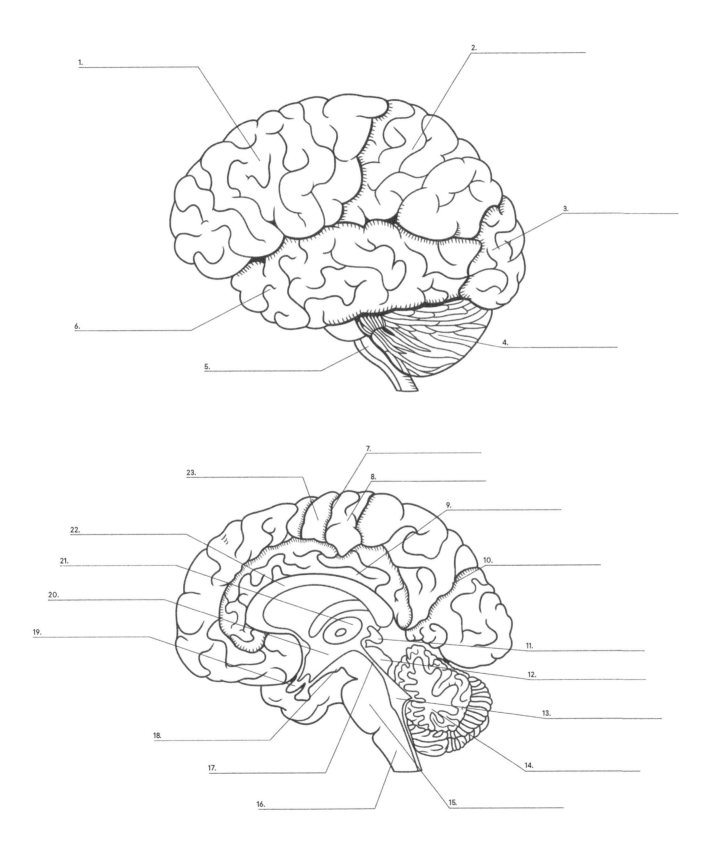

1. Frontal lobe
2. Parietal lobe
3. Occipital lobe
4. Cerebellum
5. Spinal cord
6. Temporal lobe
7. Central sulcus
8. Postcentral gyrus
9. Limbic lobe
10. Parieto-occipital sulcus
11. Pineal gland
12. Corpora quadrigemina

13. Fourth ventricle
14. Cerebellum
15. Pons
16. Medulla oblongata
17. Aqueduct of the midbrain
18. Mamillary body
19. Optic chiasm
20. Hypothalamus
21. Thalamus
22. Corpus callosum
23. Precentral gyrus

NOTES:

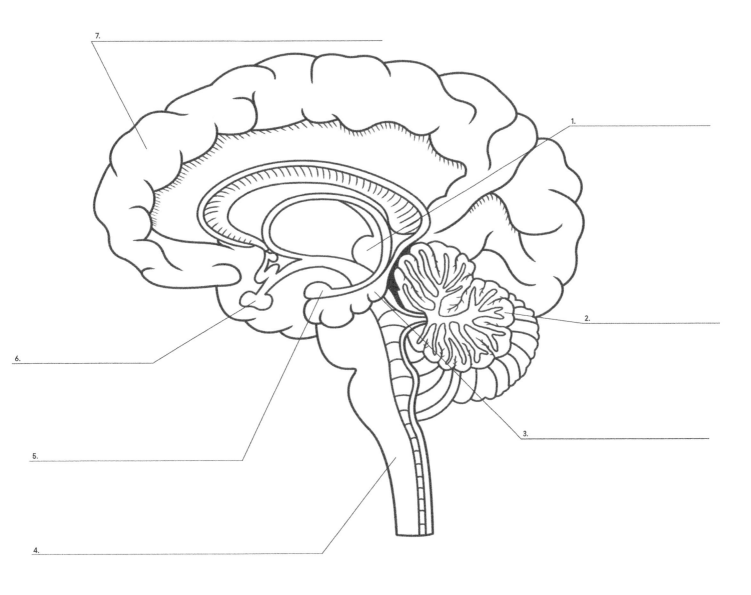

7.

1.

2.

6.

3.

5.

4.

1. Hypothalamus
2. Cerebelum
3. Hippocamous
4. Brain stem
5. Amygdala
6. Pituitary gland
7. Prefrontal corex

## NOTES:

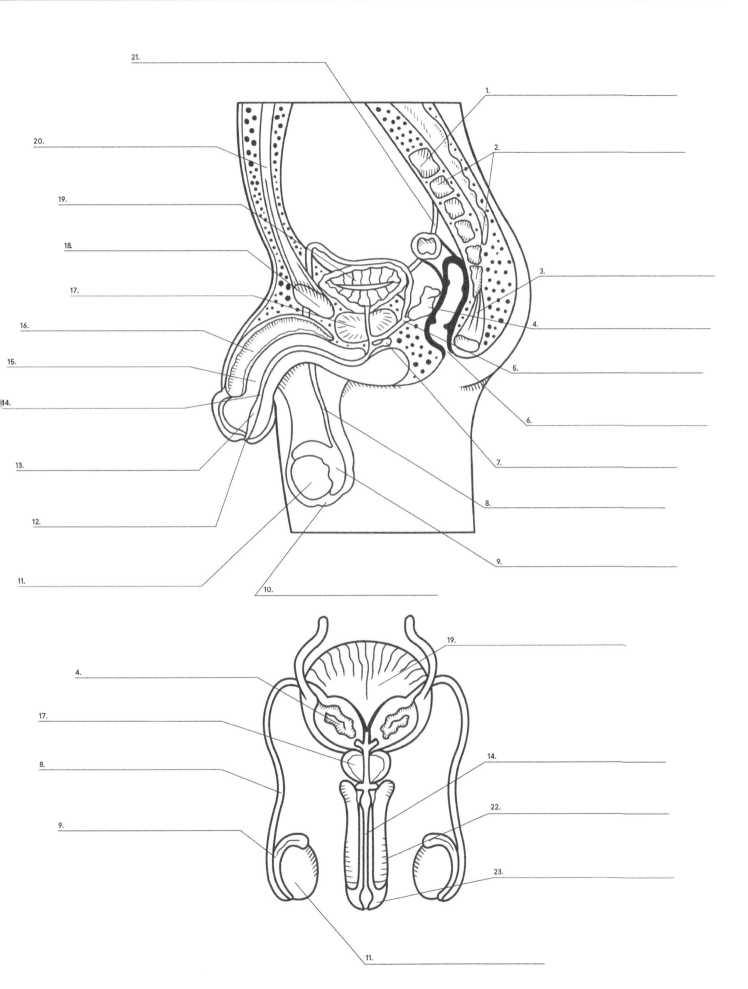

1. Sacrum bone
2. Coccyx bone
3. Pelvic floor muscles
4. Seminal vesicle
5. Ejaculatory duct
6. Anus
7. Bulbourethral gland
8. Vas deferens
9. Epididymis
10. Scrotum
11. Testicle
12. Urethral opening

13. Navicular fossa
14. Urethra
15. Corpus spongiosum
16. Corpus cavernosum
17. Prostate
18. Pubic symphysis
19. Bladder
20. Abdominal muscle
21. Ureter
22. Penis glans
23. Foreskin

## NOTES:

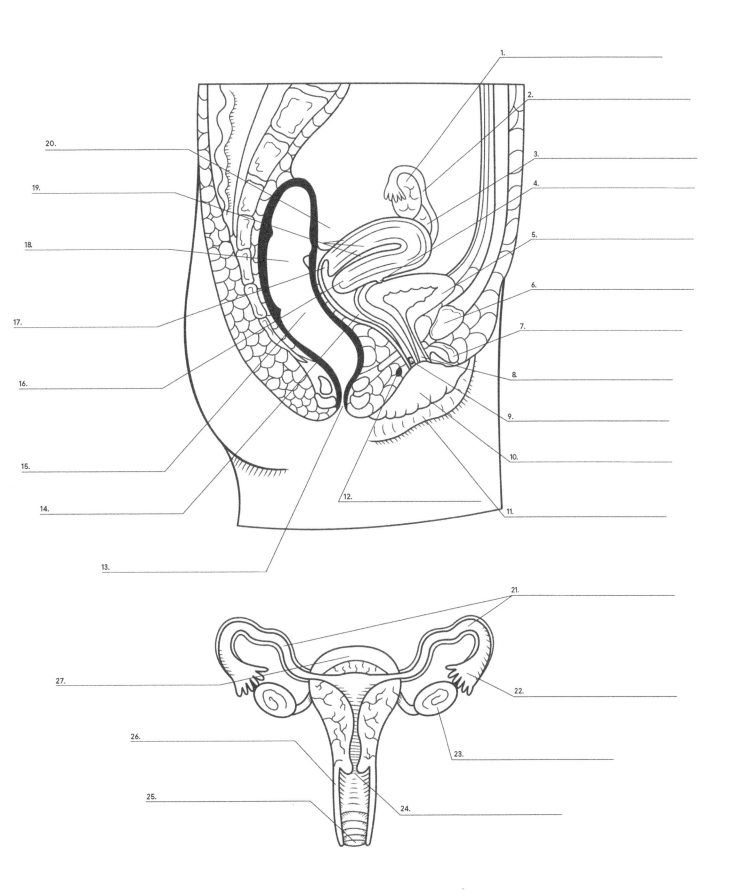

1. Ovary
2. Uterine tube
3. Broad ligament
4. Vesicouterine pouch
5. Urinary bladder
6. Pubic symphysis
7. Clitoris
8. Urethra
9. Paraurethral glands
10. Labium minus
11. Labium majus
12. Greater vestibular gland
13. Anus
14. Vagina
15. Rectum
16. Cervix
17. Fornix
18. Sigmoid colon
19. Uterus (Myometrium, Perimetrium, Endometrium)
20. Rectouterine pouch
21. Fallopian tubes
22. Fimbrae
23. Ovary
24. Cervix
25. Vaginal canal
26. Endometrium
27. Uterus

NOTES:

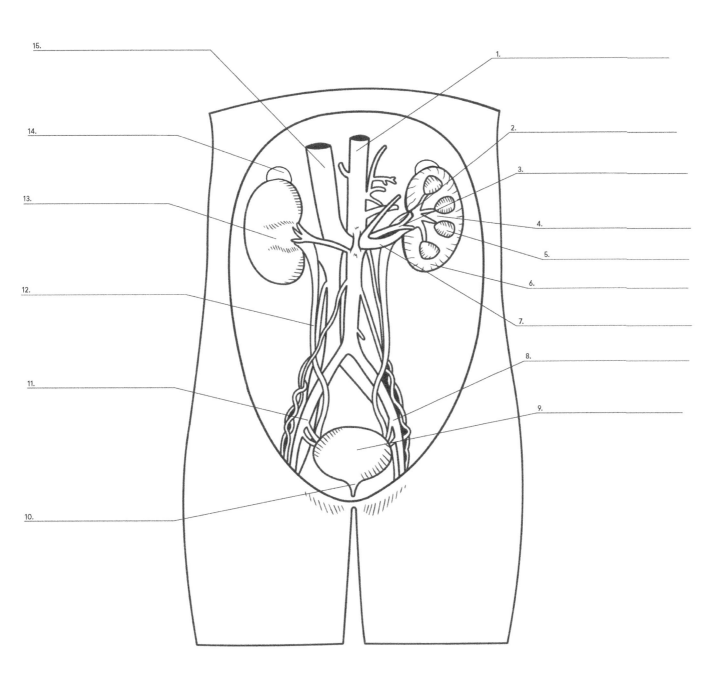

15.

14.

13.

12.

11.

10.

1.

2.

3.

4.

5.

6.

7.

8.

9.

# 11. URINARY SYSTEM

1. Descending aorta
2. Renal Pelvis
3. Renal artery
4. Renal column
5. Medullary pyramid
6. Cortex
7. Renal vein
8. Common iliac artery
9. Bladder
10. Urethra
11. Common iliac vein
12. Ureter
13. Right kidney
14. Adrenal gland
15. Inferior vena cava

## NOTES:

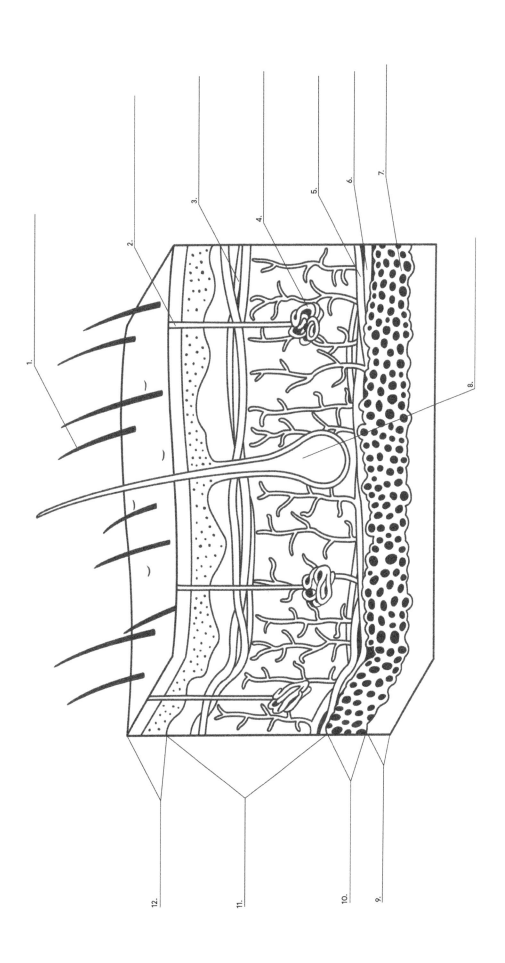

1. Hair
2. Sweet pore
3. Nerve
4. Sweat gland
5. Vein
6. Artery
7. Adipose tissue
8. Hair bulb
9. Subcutaneous layer
10. Hypodermis
11. Derma
12. Epidermis

**NOTES:**

19.

1.

2.

3.

4.

20.

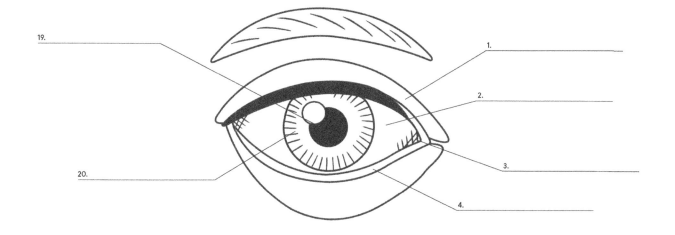

5.

6.

7.

8.

9.

10.

11.

12.

1.

2.

20.

19.

18.

17.

16.

15.

14.

13.

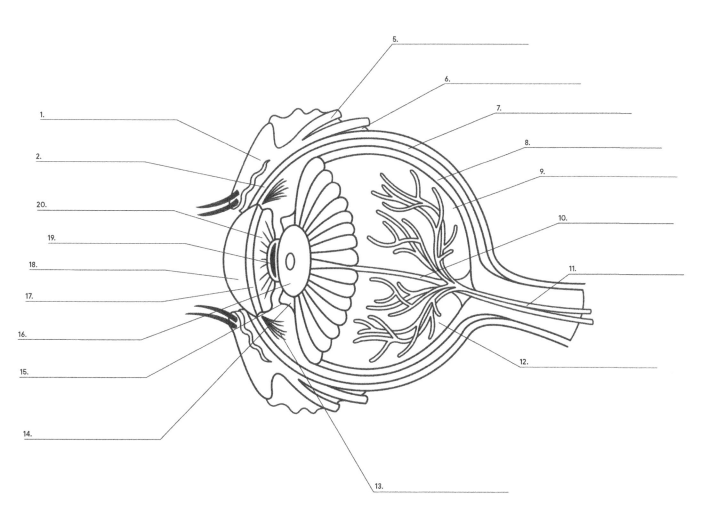

1. Eye Lid
2. Sclera
3. Lacrimal caruncle
4. Tear duct
5. Lateral rectus musce
6. Medialis rectus muscle
7. Choroid
8. Retina
9. Fovea centralis
10. Hyaloid canal

11. Optical nerve retinal blood vessels
12. Vitreous body
13. Ciliary body and muscle
14. Suspensory ligament
15. Posterior chamber
16. Lens
17. Anterior chamber
18. Cornea
19. Pupil
20. Iris

## NOTES:

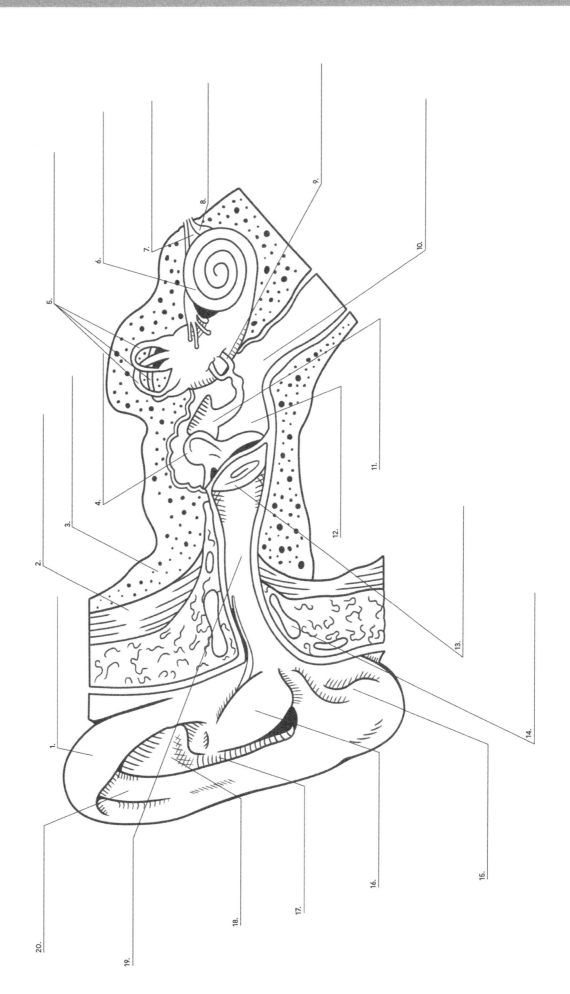

# 14. EAR ANATOMY

1. Helix
2. Temporal muscle
3. Temporal bone
4. Maiieus
5. Semicircular canals
6. Cochlea
7. Cochlear nerve
8. Vestibular nerve
9. Stapes
10. Eustachian tube
11. Incus
12. Tympanic cavity
13. Tympanic membrane (Eardrum)
14. Cartilage
15. Auricular lobule (Earlobe)
16. Concha
17. Antihelix
18. Tringular fossa
19. External acoustic meatus
20. Scapha

## NOTES:

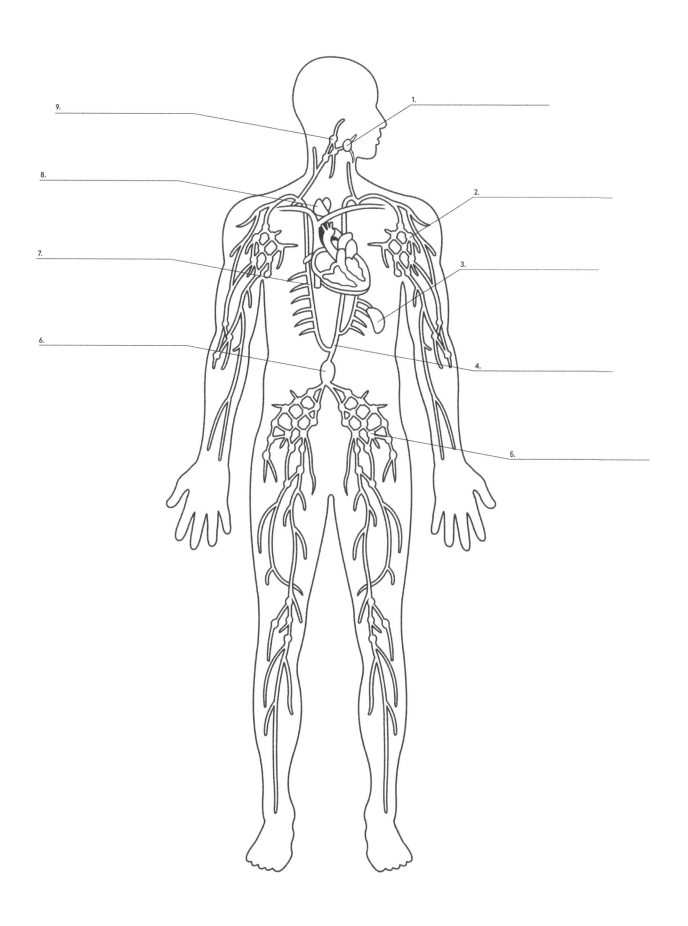

9.

1.

8.

2.

7.

3.

6.

4.

5.

1. Paladin tonsils
2. Axillary lymph nodes
3. Spleen
4. Thoracic duct
5. Inguinal lymph nodes
6. Cisterna chyli
7. Right lymphatic duct
8. Thymus
9. Cervical lymph nodes

## NOTES:

Made in the USA
Coppell, TX
28 August 2023

20878237R00039